Evidence-based Medicine for the Uninitiated

Tony Lockett
Associate Director
Health Economics
Covance

RADCLIFFE MEDICAL PRESS
OXFORD and NEW YORK

Radcliffe Medical Press Ltd
18 Marcham Road, Abingdon, Oxon OX14 1AA, UK

Radcliffe Medical Press, Inc.
141 Fifth Avenue, New York, NY 10010, USA

British Library Cataloguing in Publication Data

A catalogue record for this book is available from the British Library.

ISBN 1 85775 235 X

Library of Congress Cataloging-in-Publication Data is available.

Typeset by Acorn Bookwork, Salisbury, Wiltshire
Printed and bound by Biddles Ltd, Guildford and King's Lynn

Contents

Preface

In 1969, the first trials on the effectiveness of streptokinase in reducing the effects of myocardial infarction were described. The effectiveness of thrombolysins is now well known. However, currently fewer than 30% of patients in a UK hospital, who are eligible for such treatments, receive them. This has a considerable impact on costs, and mortality of patients. It is a pattern which is being repeated in many medical practices across the world. Known effective interventions are not being used – or worse still, interventions that are known to cause patients physical harm are being held in high esteem.

In studies of medical decision-making, current practice was described by the group of Macmaster researchers as follows:[1]

- unsystematic observations of clinical practice provided a valid way of building professional knowledge about the progression of disease, the value of diagnostic tests and the method of treatment
- the study of basic pathophysiology provided information on the clinical behaviour of patients
- there was no need for traditional medical training to provide details of how to evaluate diagnostic tests and treatments, as clinical practice and pathologic understanding enabled the validity of a system to be understood
- continued medical practice provided sufficient exposure to permit skill development.

This paradigm of medical decision-making has been labelled as 'muddling through elegantly'. This method of medical decision-making has been labelled as causing the great variations in medical practice across the health care services. For example, the rates of hysterectomy operations can vary as much as 100-fold between neighbouring health districts.

Faced with these problems, action has been demanded to place medical decision-making on a more solid footing, in a manner that is both understandable and defensible. In response to this call for action, we have seen the evolution of evidence-based medicine and cost-effective medicine. These methods are not new. They represent an extension of techniques used in other industries and ideologies. Therefore, evidence-based medicine is seen as an extension of the scientific method, while cost-effectiveness based decision-making is a reflection of the tools used in economic theory. The fact that these tools are imported into medical practice means that inevitably there will be some conflict between the paradigms of the decision-making processes and the practice of medicine, and indeed this is the case. It is the aim of this text to highlight the discussions and explore the current ideas on how best to structure medical decision-making, pointing out, wherever possible, the benefits and limitations of the methods proposed.

The book is divided into four parts, each of which is designed to be self-standing. Part I explores the possible routes by which medical decision-making can be reformed, focusing on the levers that can be applied. It also seeks to set the stage for the introduction of evidence-based and cost-effective decision-making models.

Part II focuses specifically on evidence-based medicine.

Part III focuses on cost-effectiveness based medical decision-making.

Finally, Part IV debates the balance that should be achieved between the various models of decision-making currently being employed.

The overall objective of the book is to host and facilitate an informed debate about the new paradigms of medical decision-making. It is based in part on its forebear *Health economics for the uninitiated*,[2] but also on the discussions I have had with medical decision-makers and those interested in the subject of rationing and decision-making.

As with the previous volume, all comments are welcome.

Tony Lockett
October 1996

References

1. The Evidence-based Medicine Working Group (1992) Evidence-based medicine: a new approach to teaching the practice of medicine. *JAMA.* **268**(17): 2420–5.
2. Lockett T (1996) *Health economics for the uninitiated.* Radcliffe Medical Press, Oxford.

Part I   Introduction

1 The levers of decision-making in medical practice

> *Key points*
>
> *The current paradigm of medical decision-making – labelled as 'muddling through elegantly' – is based on the unique knowledge of the individual physician about medical practice. It is characterized by applying pathophysiological-based enquiry to individual patients.*
>
> *The method has been criticized for leading to the situation where there are large variations in medical practice. Patients sometimes receive ineffective, or poorly effective, treatment. In response to these concerns, alternative decision-making criteria have been proposed – evidence-based decision-making and cost-effective decision-making. These two methods build on the experiences of decision-makers outside health care and therefore there is some controversy about their application.*

Decision-making requires a substrate to work. In the case of health care the substrate is the framework that supports health care and the viewpoint of the individuals within that framework. With this in mind, Part I seeks to review the fundamental forces shaping health care decision-making, and apply them to the development of the new decision-making paradigms.

Why does health care exist?

This is not as odd a question as it might seem at first. It is part of human nature to care; in a manner that benefits both ourselves

3

Table 1.1 Summary of choice faced by the health authority

Treatment	A	B
Success : treated ratio	1 : 6	1 : 4
Cost per treatment	£600	£1500
Number treated	38	12
Babies	5	3

and others. This apparently simple situation hides a paradox. Is it the role of health care to offer care to the individual, or to offer care to as many patients as possible, given scarce resources? The nature of this paradox is best explained by an example.

Consider two treatments, A and B, for infertility, being considered by a health authority which has £18 000 to spend. The choice faced by the health authority is summarized in Table 1.1.

If the health authority acts in the best interest of the individual, i.e. acts to assure the most possible chance for the individual to conceive, then it would select treatment B. However, this would result in fewer babies and fewer treatments from a society viewpoint. If, in contrast, the aim of the health authority is to maximize the benefits of health care to society, then it would choose treatment A, even though it lessened the individual's chance of conceiving.

In making decisions, therefore, the division is absolute; either an individual-based decision or a society-based decision is made. This dichotomy of decisions has been summarized as the dichotomy between the greatest good for the greatest number (often termed utilitarianism), or the greatest good for the individual (often termed libertarianism). It is very clear that whichever decision-making framework is chosen, it has a profound influence on how decisions are made. Accordingly, there is great debate about the merits of either system.

Utilitarianists postulate that the greater benefit to society must be at the centre of all welfare states and that it is the government's right to decide the greater number to be treated (if you like, it is the role of the government to decide the social order and ranking of suffering). However, libertarians argue that suffering can only be assessed on the individual level and that the government's role is to set the boundaries of the services provided. In practice, it is possible to design a decision-making process and indeed an entire health care system using either utilitarianism or libertarianism, but in either case the distortions of the system must be accepted.

In utilitarian-based systems the suffering of the individual is placed second to society. We have seen this situation with the case of child B,[1] where the judge's ruling was that it was correct for the health authority to withhold treatment, given the benefit that could be obtained for others in society from the funds it would take to treat the leukaemia from which the child was suffering. Under this ethic, however, it might mean that if the majority of the population were smokers, then treatment should be offered to these individuals instead of those with rarer conditions (the so-called perverse taste paradox).

The libertarian view places benefit to the individual above that of society. It is the view taken by many general practitioners in the UK – who view their role as to secure health for the patient in front of them. The libertarian view could, if applied, mean that those who have great suffering that is self-inflicted, may take precedence over those with genetic disorders.

From this discussion it is apparent that both systems of health care have been, and are, applied. However, both have potential problems (more of which will be discussed later in this book). The new paradigms of medical decision-making have root in these two systems. Evidence-based medicine is most synonymous with the benefit for the individual patient, while decision analysis has root in utilitarian policy. However – as we will discuss later – it is not as clear-cut as the statement suggests.

Information and levers for change

For any new decision-making process to work, both information and levers are needed. In the case of health services the two are intrinsically linked. The levers for change in medical decision-making have been classified as information which provides evidence for:

- *Professional change.* This includes evidence for the effectiveness of procedures, the effects of guidelines and the integrity of professional values. The application of professional levers also includes the use of audit and other performance measures based on process and outcome. These levers are the aim of evidence-based medicine and, to an extent, cost–benefit associated medicine. They are difficult to apply correctly, as we will see, but are a major focus.

- *Customer change.* This includes the satisfaction of patients, the understanding of patients about treatments, and the acceptability of treatment to patients. This is a difficult set of levers for change to apply. It is difficult, first, to define who the customers are, and second, to define who takes responsibility. This aspect is covered in greater detail in Part IV.

- *Economic levers.* These include the use of financial information to shift ideas and purchasing, and the use of contracting mechanisms. In the past the strength of financial levers has been over-emphasized. The strength of financial leverage depends on the amount of free, and freeable, funding available. However, studies have shown that the amount of uncommitted moneys may be small. In this circumstance the emphasis shifts to efficiency and demand management, both of which have a heavy professional input.

The limitation of the levers we have mentioned explains why there is a focus on the use of professional levers via evidence-based medicine and cost-effective medicine. However, as we will discuss, the application of these levers is problematical without a clear definition of the purpose of medical practice.

The nature of the levers and the process of rationing

The decision-making process, together with the levers applied, enables a description of the processes in rationing. These processes are important from a philosophical and ethical viewpoint, as any one of them can be used to make a viable resource allocation system. The impact of these processes is the subject of the remainder of this book.

Resource allocation systems may be:

- technocratic – where the professionals' values and beliefs decide who benefits from health care
- bureaucratic – where the process of government decides who benefits from health care
- market-based – where economic factors decide the distribution of health care
- democratic – where the values of society decide the distribution of benefit.

The current emphasis on cost-effectiveness and evidence-based medicine drives – for reasons that will become apparent – a technocratic process.

Summary

The limitations of our ability to manage financial levers or construct customer-based tools implies that decision-making is driven by professional values. This explains why there is an emphasis on evidence-based and cost-effective medicine. The use of professional levers tends to make the decision-making processes technocratic, with a bias towards utilitarianism.

In order to minimize the possible effects that these processes may have on medical practice, it is important that the reasons why and the purposes of the decision under scrutiny are reviewed.

Reference

1. Entwhistle V, Bradbury R, Pehl L *et al.* (1996) Media coverage of the Child B case. *BMJ*. **312**: 1587–90.

Part II Evidence-based Medicine

2 Evidence-based medicine

> **Key points from the previous chapter**
>
> *Our limited understanding of medical decision-making tools forces us to consider professional decision-making tools. Two are proposed: evidence-based medicine and cost-effectiveness associated medicine. Both of these techniques are borrowed from other disciplines and are prone to cause distortion in the health care system.*

Part II covers the basic aspects of evidence-based medicine (relating to its definition and practice) and its tangible effects.

An introduction to evidence-based medicine

Evidence-based medicine: panacea or the frontier of medical science; the effective use of managerialism or the decline of the medical profession? What is it actually?

Evidence-based medicine (EBM) is the product of a long tradition of the medical model and rationality in medicine. As such, there are serious questions to be asked about a medical model-based health care system in the practice of modern social medicine.

Evidence-based medicine is a much flaunted term. New definitions and interpretations appear almost weekly – or so it seems. However, for the purposes of this book the author wishes to define EBM as the process of systematically finding, appraising, and using contemporaneous research findings as a basis for clinical decisions. This definition gives us the aim of EBM: 'The aim of evidence-based medicine is to eliminate the use of expensive, ineffective, or dangerous medical decision-making.[1]

The paradigm of decision-making under EBM is ensuring the most effective care for the individual. However, in doing so it relies on the evidence derived from populations, a paradox that does cause some problems, as we will see later.

The ideas behind EBM are not new. All clinicians consult the literature, at least occasionally. However, EBM makes explicit the desire to feature the use of published literature in decision-making.

Evidence-based medicine is a product of the information age. Its application is technology dependent and co-exists with the development of information systems. The existence of relatively inexpensive data retrieval systems and computers has lessened the costs of making information available, and harnessing it – through protocols – for medical and clinical practice. The trends towards EBM have been enhanced by the new managerialism and emphasis on rationality in health services. The application of managerial techniques to the management of medicine is apparent in many health care systems. The joining together of information and management tools is a common theme in many changes impacting society, so much so, that the term *information culture* is now used. However, the unique nature of health care makes it very susceptible to the influence of information, with possibly disastrous results.

Reference

1. Rosenberg W and Donald A (1995) Evidence-based medicine: an approach to clinical problem-solving. *BMJ.* **310**: 1122–6.

3 The history of evidence-based medicine

> *Key points from the previous chapter*
>
> *Evidence-based medicine makes explicit the use of research findings to guide medical practice. In this way it hopes to eliminate much of the waste and danger associated with medical therapy.*

Chapter 3 reviews evidence-based medicine from an historical viewpoint, together with an understanding of why it has developed.

The development of clinical trial methods

The development of the EBM model for the management of medical care has paralleled the development of clinical trials. However, it is only since clinical trial methods have been established that EBM approaches have become applicable.

Louis, in 1834, elaborated the 'numerical method' for assessing treatments.[1] He advocated the need for exact observations of treatment, the definitions of disease, the knowledge of the progression of disease, and the recording of deviations from intended treatments. His first application of these methods was in a study of the treatment of pneumonia by bleeding. Louis was immensely influential outside of his native Paris and found favour in Britain and the USA. For example, Lister used the numerical method in developing an effective antiseptic technique. However, it was not until the mid-twentieth century that significant advances in clinical trial design were achieved. For example, 'blinding' patients and doctors – so that neither knew which drugs were being administered – was introduced in 1917, and randomization (randomly assigning patients to treatment and control groups) was introduced in 1948. However, it is since 1950 that randomized controlled clinical trials have become the vogue. This is led by drug standards with regard to safety, quality, and efficacy, required for the registration of new pharmaceutical products.

The need for the stringent control of the registration of pharmaceutical products arose as a result of the thalidomide disaster in 1961; where a medicine was released on to the market without adequate safety assessments being considered. Since 1963 there has been a requirement for clinical trials prior to a market licence being granted. The introduction of good clinical practice guidelines in the 1980s further strengthened the position of clinical trials in drug development.

The gap between clinical trials and clinical practice

Despite the development of rigorous clinical trial methods, it became apparent that there is a gap between the results of randomized, blinded clinical studies and the practical use of the treatments in the usual clinical setting. The problems in this area are exemplified by the introduction of thrombolysins for the management of myocardial infarction where, as was mentioned in the Preface, fewer than 30% of patients receive this life-saving therapy. It was instances such as this which prompted the explicit use of information to drive medical practice.

The development of evidence-based medicine

Faced with the problems in using clinical trial information to influence medical practice, a group of investigators at the Macmaster University in Ontario, Canada, set out to understand the current model for medical decision-making and substitute a new paradigm that would be more flexible in relation to the information made available from clinical trials. They termed this new paradigm *evidence-based medicine*. In contrast to the model of 'muddling through elegantly', the new model can be classified in the following way:

- clinical experience and instincts are crucial to practising medicine, and many areas of clinical practice remain unquestioned and unchallenged. However, there is a need to record clinical experience in an unbiased and reproducible fashion, and in such a manner that a body of knowledge may be acquired that will aid the description of the patient's prognosis
- the study of pathophysiology is not a sufficient basis for understanding disease
- clinical information should be subject to rules of evidence to enable the diagnosis and treatment of a disease to be evaluated correctly, by a clinician and also in the literature.

The new paradigm makes explicit the scenario that the clinician is able to critically appraise and use the evidence to provide optimal treatment care. It also places much more of an emphasis on the individual doctor and less on the role of experts.

Summary

The development of evidence-based medicine occurred at a very propitious time. The continuing rise in health care expenditure is a 'hot' topic. Evidence-based medicine offers a mechanism by which the available expenditure could be better distributed by clinical belief. It is therefore an idea of its age and has been readily accepted. The role of EBM and management will be discussed later in this book, but EBM has now become one of the major catchphrases in the development of modern medicine.

Reference

1. Louis P (1835) *Recherche sur les effets de la Siagnée*. De Mignaret, Paris.

Further reading

Pocock SJ (1983) *Clinical trials – a practical approach.* Wiley and Sons, Chichester.

The Evidence-based Medicine Working Group (1992) Evidence-based medicine: a new approach to teaching the practice of medicine. *JAMA.* **268**: 2420–5.

4 The practicalities of evidence-based medicine

> **Key points from the previous chapter**
>
> *Evidence-based medicine aims to make health care better by closing a perceived gap in the practical application of proven medical interventions and by the development of rationally communicated clinical experiences used to guide medical practice. This also requires the departure from the pathophysiologic models of medicine. The development of EBM coincided with changes in the role of medical practice and in the health care delivery systems, that have made its uptake easier.*

This chapter reviews the practical aspects of evidence-based medicine and how to introduce it into a clinical setting. The process of EBM can be broken down into several clear steps.

Posing the question

Questions are key to the process of developing an evidence-based approach. Without them it is impossible to find the needed evidence or appraise the results. The questions asked can relate to the diagnosis, treatment, quality or economics of care. Questions should be specific, and to be formulated must take into consideration:

- the type of patient, e.g. uncomplicated diabetics, aged 22–45
- the nature of the intervention, e.g. six-monthly retinal screening

- the outcome desired, e.g. the prevention of blindness.

For example, suitable questions from the above examples could be:

- what is the risk of developing blindness in uncomplicated diabetics, aged 22–45?
  or
- what is the reduction in the risk of blindness as a result of diabetes if uncomplicated diabetics, aged 22–45, have retinal screening every six months?

Finding the evidence

Once the question is formulated then the evidence to support the question is needed. This requires the searching of databases. Two types of databases are apparent. First, there are the biblio-graphic sources, such as Medline. These are databases that permit the identification of citations based on bibliographic terms – authors, keywords, titles, and alike. These databases are relatively cheap but are very dependent upon the search strate-gies used to generate the bibliography. In one recent study of the validation of a Medline search, carried out by librarian staff, over 30% of key references were found to be missing when compared with a manual search. The concern over bibliographic searches has led to the generation of so-called publication-based databases, where the primary source of the data is made directly available. The Cochrane Database of Systematic Reviews is one example. These databases do not, however, alleviate the problems associated with Medline searching. Medline is often used to identify the initial article.

Appraising the evidence

Once the data has been collected then its quality must be appraised. The screens that are applied to appraise data have been summarized as critical appraisal methods. Several templates have been designed to do this. In general, these templates rely on asking questions on the material presented. These questions, while seeming simple, require some mastery as their application is not straightforward. A typical set of questions is reproduced below.

Critical appraisal questions[1,2]

Are the results valid?

- Was the assignment of treatment to patients randomized?
- Were all patients entered into the trial accounted for?
- Was follow-up complete?
- Were the patients' results analysed in accordance with the groups they were randomized to?
- Were the health workers and patients blinded to the treatment used?
- Were the groups similar at the start of the trial?
- Aside from the intervention, were the groups studied treated equally?

What was the result?

- How large was the treatment effect?
- How precise was the treatment effect?

Will the results impact care for my patients?

- Can the results be applied?
- Were all the outcomes considered?
- Are the benefits worth the potential costs?

Significant training must be applied to the application of these questions, for although written in common language, their use relates to the so-called rules of evidence. Particular care must be taken in the following points.

Ensuring the results are valid

The development of EBM places a distinct hierarchy on the

value of evidence. The most valid results are those from randomized, controlled clinical trials, followed by uncontrolled trials, cohort studies and lastly, case reports. The hierarchy of evidence is not without challenge. Controlled clinical trials are often restrictive in the patients they recruit, and cohort studies reflect a more normal patient management pattern. This debate is far from resolved.

Determining the size of the treatment effect

The results of clinical trials are often dichotomous in that patients are classified as alive or dead at the end of the trial – a major example of this is cancer trials. Information of this type requires careful interpretation as to whether the treatment effect was sufficiently large to justify the use of the intervention. There are many ways in which a dichotomous treatment effect can be expressed. One method is the determination of the absolute risk reduction; that is the proportion of patients who died in each treatment group minus the proportion that died in the control group. This method is determinate on the size of the groups in question and in response the relative risk reduction (RRR) is the more quoted measure. This is defined as:

$$RRR = 1 - x/y$$

where x and y are the properties of the selected 'outcomes' of treatments in each group. For example: in a trial, the proportion of deaths under one treatment is 0.15 (x) and 0.20 (y), the absolute risk reduction was 0.05 (0.2–0.15) while the RRR was 0.25 or 25%. The second figure is easier to interpret as patients under the first treatment had a 25% reduction in the chance of death.

How precise was the determination of the treatment effect?

When calculating the risk reduction it should be borne in mind that the true risk reduction cannot be known; all we achieve from clinical trials is an estimate of the risk reduction. The range of values for the RRR can be statistically estimated using the calculation of confidence intervals (CI).

The calculation of confidence intervals involves an estimation of the $\pm 95\%$ range for the point value of the RRR. The choice of a 95% range is somewhat arbitrary and relates closely to the concept of statistical significance. The value of the CI range reflects the fact that 95 times out of 100 the RRR will lie within this range. The selection of this significance level is largely unquestioned by many of the proponents of EBM. The origin of this level of significance ($p < 0.05$) has its roots in the philosophy of Kurt Gödel. Gödel was concerned at the level of proof required to define a certain value within a formal mathematical system. That is, he was concerned with questions of mathematical truth in systems where the final answer cannot be known, either due to the complexity of the problem or the magnitude of the numbers involved. His solution was to examine the consistency of the result and to determine a level of consistency by which the propositions of mathematical proofs could be said to be true. His work was used by the early statisticians to determine the consistency of the statistical results that determine the truth of a statement. As a direct result of these deliberations the $p < 0.05$ benchmark was adopted. However, many individuals question the validity of these assumptions.

When working with confidence intervals it should be remembered that calculations of this type are very sensitive to sample size. In general, the larger the trial the smaller the confidence interval. Therefore, in small trials with dramatic results, there may be insufficient evidence to justify the use of the procedure.

Despite the drawbacks, the principle of a confidence interval analysis adds significantly to the power to analyse trials. If a confidence interval includes zero or is minus (for example a confidence interval of -38% or -50%) then the treatment potentially gives the patient no benefit, and may even cause harm. The range of confidence interval also gives the opportunity to judge whether the effect is clinically significant. For example, in a cancer trial the CI for the RRR was estimated as

2–4%. This can be judged as a very small benefit in the face of cost.

One of the problems in using confidence intervals is that very few papers actually quote them. Instead they must be estimated. Quite often with the aid of a statistician experienced in these methods, this can be done. However, two quick rules include:

1. where the p value = 0.05, the lower limit of the CI must be zero. Therefore when $p < 0.05$ the trial always has a positive effect
2. where a standard error (SE) is quoted, the CI is roughly twice the SE.

Assessing if the results apply to the patients in question

The first step in seeking to use the trial result is to review the inclusion/exclusion criteria applied to the recruitment of the individuals included in the analysis of the study. If the patient or patient population violates any of the criteria then the results must be interpreted with caution. In these situations it is up to the judgement of the clinician as to whether the deviation invalidates the results.

A word of caution should be injected here. It has been the vogue to perform subgroup analysis, particularly where there is doubt over the magnitude of the treatment effect. These subgroup analyses are very prone to data effects, particularly when the sample size gets small. Therefore, using subgroup analysis to decide treatments must be carefully managed. Small differences in subgroup population benefits are generally best ignored. However, when it was the intention to perform a subgroup analysis when the study started – or in studies where the number of subgroups is very small – then subgroup analysis can be useful.

Were all important outcomes considered?

Treatments should be considered if, and only if, they offer significant benefit. But what is a benefit? A slight improvement in lung function as a result of an improved bronchodilator may be statistically significant – but the question remains, is it representative of an improved outcome? For an improved outcome, a decrease in shortness of breath is required or an improved exercise tolerance. However, as these are often difficult to quantify, substitute endpoints are often used. In these cases it is important to understand the relation between the substitute endpoint and the final outcome. The classic example of this was the use of depolarizing agents (such as flecainide) for post-myocardial infarction. The suppression of arrhythmias was used as a substitute endpoint in the early studies as it was supposed that suppressing arrhythmias would lessen cardiac deaths. Indeed, the studies showed that the use of these drugs did indeed suppress arrhythmias. However, subsequent studies displayed the fact that this was not a good endpoint, and in fact the number of deaths increased with the use of flecainide after myocardial infarction.

Caution must be used, even with clinically important endpoints. When reporting a favourable outcome, the temptation is to ignore the effect on other outcomes. The recent controversy over the increase in non-cardiac deaths as a result of lipid-lowering drugs is a good example. In the final analysis, like the view about the size of the effect of treatment, the discussion about relevant outcomes is a subjective opinion. However, the guides expanded upon above may assist the decision-maker.

Are the benefits worth the costs?

This is the crucial question. A 25% reduction in mortality may sound impressive – but is it worth the total 'cost' of treatment? A useful concept to assist this evaluation is the number needed to treat (NNT) and the number needed to harm (NNH).

An assessment of the NNT and NNH provides an easy way to determine the total picture of the effect of a treatment. As we have seen the RRR, while valuable as a statistical concept, is not readily understandable. The NNT and NNH, however, convert relative risk into a lay expression. These measures encompass the concept of the RRR but use the metric of 'people treated' to convey the message.

The NNT is calculated by inverting the absolute risk reduction as a result of treatment. As an example, consider the use of beta-blockers. These drugs reduce the risk of myocardial infarction in hypertensive subjects by 25%. This equates to a risk reduction of 25% or 0.0025. The inverse of this is 400. Therefore 400 patients are treated to see one patient benefiting.

The NNH is allied to this concept. Consider the adverse event of fatigue associated with the use of beta-blockers. In this case, the risk of fatigue is increased to 10%. Therefore one in every ten patients will complain of fatigue. Applying this to the figures used above, 400 patients are needed to avert one myocardial infarction, while 40 will suffer from fatigue. This statement gives a risk–benefit assessment that can be used to subjectively assess the treatment in question. When costs are attached to the NNT and NNH ratios, a subjective assessment of the value of the treatment becomes possible. For example, if the cost of treating 400 patients equals the cost of one hip replacement, then the benefit of the hip and the one patient who benefits from the beta-blocker treatment become comparable. However, this comparison is subject to the same difficulties as experienced with quality adjusted life years (QALYs). Both of these assessments rely on the individual making the assessment to express a preference. In the case of QALYs this effect has led to the methodology falling into disrepute.

Acting on the evidence

Having 'valued' the presented evidence, it must then be acted upon. This is the most difficult aspect of EBM. All of the reviews conducted so far suggest that doctors cling to preconceived ideas and the best way in which to effect change in medical practice has yet to be found. Recent reviews have suggested that change may best be achieved by the use of clinically-oriented discussion groups reviewing the evidence and then discussing it. This is a skilful exercise and it is difficult to achieve in general practice where the vast majority of clinical care takes place.

Summary

This section has reviewed the subject of the practical application of the ideology of evidence-based medicine. The current weakness in EBM must be the lack of research into its use, in particular the statistical validity of the methods used, and how best to influence the behaviours of doctors. Despite this, the practice of EBM is having an impact on medical practice. The effects of EBM on the conduct of medicine is the subject of the next chapter.

References

1. Oxman D, Sacklett D and Guyatt G (1993) User's guide to the medical literature: getting started. *JAMA.* **270**: 2093–5.
2. Guyatt G, Sacklett D and Cook D (1994) User's guide to the medical literature: how to use an article. *JAMA.* **271**: 59–63.

5 The effects of evidence-based medicine

Key points from the previous chapter

Evidence-based medicine relies on the use of a structured appraisal method to determine the value of any research conducted and the resultant publications. The effect of EBM is therefore very dependent on the methods used to search and appraise articles and how the results are applied. While there is a great deal of research into the retrieval and appraisal of articles, less emphasis has been placed on its practical use.

Evidence-based medicine raises a number of issues. In particular, how effective is it? What are the ethical, political and managerial issues? Finally, what are the effects on patient care in the holistic sense? This chapter is a practical introduction to these issues.

Appraising the appraiser – how to quantify the effects of evidence-based medicine

The term evidence-based medicine, like every catchphrase, has a tendency to be overused and applied like a label to anything that remotely resembles the concept or is new. Furthermore, as EBM is a process rather than an outcome ('the patient had four evidence-based units of improvement, doctor') it should be measured by both process and outcome measures. These features make the appraisal of EBM difficult, but not impossible! But before deciding that EBM is a radical concept and therefore embracing it (or not), we have to examine the current situation about the level to which clinical practice is already evidence-based. This will assist us in determining what is to be appraised and also the scale on which we are to appraise it.

Evidence-based decisions are used in clinical practice

In studies conducted in routine clinical settings it has been shown that many decisions made by doctors can be supported by clinical evidence. Those areas shown to be less evidence-based tend to be the super-specialties and research facilities. If these results are accepted then EBM can be appraised on the basis of improving clinical decision-making, that is, improving the number of patients who received EBM-based care, and the metric becomes the outcomes of therapy in treated patients and the time taken to reach decisions. This scheme covers process (time) and outcome measures. This is, in fact, what has happened. Articles appear weekly in the medical press claiming that this treatment regimen improves outcome over another. Taken at face value these reports appear valuable. However, there is another side to this equation. Clinical trials often exclude patients because they do not fit the protocol or refuse informed consent or were just not asked! Perhaps another metric is to look at the effects on patients who were not treated and ascertain what happened to this group. In a bygone era of the Poor Law and the pauper in England, it was common to include the drunkard and the very poor in the category of people not to be helped, as there was no evidence that they could be helped. It was not until the extreme effects of this policy became apparent that action was demanded, with dramatic results. Therefore, in the performance of clinical trials, the numbers of patients excluded becomes an important measure. The debate about the metric used to measure EBM has profound consequences on the effects of EBM. This debate includes the ethical and political dimensions of EBM, as well as its clinical effects.

The effect on clinical practice

There have been few reviews which have looked at the effects of evidence-based medicine in clinical practice. The reviews that have been conducted give a mixed picture as to its benefits. Evidence-based medicine has been shown to increase the outcome of screening procedures. However, the effect on patient care in more complex situations has not been published. In fairness, there are many reasons for this. First, EBM is a recent innovation and, second, the status of our current methodologies to assess outcomes is lacking. These problems are coupled with the uncertainty about its implementation. However, the lack of evidence about the clinical effectiveness of EBM is disappointing.

In the investigations into EBM that have been conducted a common set of problems has been encountered. Foremost of these is the time taken to learn and practise the critical skills needed. Also investigators have commented on the fact that researching a problem can take several hours and communicating it to the relevant staff even longer.

The ability to perform EBM is not without cost, as the provision of modems and subscriptions to on-line services can be expensive. This is in addition to the opportunity cost of having a full-time clinician searching a database – often ineffectively.

Even when the time, staff and facilities are available there remains a problem with the evidence found. First, medical journals tend to only publish positive results. Second, it is not uncommon to miss these results when searching as the key words used are obscure and the interface with the technology is often reported to be daunting. Where the evidence is available and of good quality, attempts to introduce the techniques have often been clumsy and led to claims of cookbook medicine and medical practices that do not encompass patient preferences for care. This concern is allied to the feeling that purchasers and managers may try and use evidence-based guises to control costs.

Taken together, it is difficult to have a cost–benefit ratio for evidence-based medicine. The lack of this only emphasizes the need to construct carefully the methods by which it is introduced.

Medical education

One of the major benefits claimed by evidence-based medicine is its potential for influencing and improving medical education. Controlled trials have shown that evidence-based methods improve the decision-making skills of medical students and integrate the students more rapidly into clinical practice. The effect this may or may not have on clinical outcomes is unknown – but it has not stopped EBM being hailed as one of the major advances in education.

Summary

The effects of EBM are difficult to quantify, although they have been hailed as a major advance. There is some suggestion that a considerable amount of clinical practice, while not being evidence-based, will stand up to evidence-testing.

Trials of EBM require long-term follow-up and large numbers of patients. Also, the ethics of construction of a clinical trial and EBM must be questionable. Is it ethical to randomize patients to evidence-based and non-evidence-based treatments? Instead of proceeding down this path it might be better to first establish the factors we should measure EBM against. These should include the ethical effects and the possible damaging effects EBM may have on the distribution of health care.

Further reading

The problems associated with the nature of scientific evidence are not just found in medicine. For an interesting debate see *Cordelia's Dilemma* in Gould SJ (1996) *Dinosaurs in a haystack*. Jonathan Cape, London.

6 Ethics, philosophy and evidence-based medicine

> **Key points from the previous chapter**
>
> *Evidence for the effects of evidence-based medicine is difficult to generate. There have been many attempts to quantify the effects, but these have mostly proved to be negative. In an attempt to look at EBM, surrogate markers are needed such as philosophical or ethical objectives.*

The need to examine in detail the possible detrimental effects of EBM stems from the way in which it looks at the world. This chapter explores the outlook on EBM and explains why it gives cause for concern.

Thought systems

Evidence-based medicine is an extension of the empirical system of thought and falls into a category containing positivism. This is a philosophy embraced by, among others, Bertrand Russell and the Vienna Circle. It is a product of twentieth-century thought and is among one of the most controversial thought systems proposed during this century.

Taken at its simplest, the positivist creed states that: 'Only those thoughts and actions that can be based on sensory evidence can be considered as true of reflecting reality'.[1] Taken at its extreme, positivism excludes all metaphysical ideas – including the existence of God and pain. This is the position adopted by the logical positivists of the Vienna Circle. However, it is generally regarded that this view is discredited. Instead, more moderate views – such as those of Ayer[2] – are adopted, in which metaphysical concepts are thought of as secondary systems within the whole.

The ideas of positivism seek to extend the principles applied during scientific experimentation to a wider range of human existence. However, philosophers such as Thomas Kuhn[3] and Karl Popper[4], have called into question if the so-called 'scientific method' exists at all. According to the classical model of scientific development, theories are developed which are changed on the basis of experimental evidence. Therefore scientific development is incremental by nature – taking small steps that accumulate. Kuhn, in his *The structure of scientific revolutions*, emphasizes that this is not the case and the way in which individual scientists behave has a great influence on the progression of science. Popper, while also dismissing the scientific method, proposes a different mechanism – that of the falsificationist – that is, theories are not modified until proven false; until this point more and more evidence is sought to verify the principle. It is widely recognized that both Kuhn and Popper suggest that scientific development is not incremental in the way positivists would have us believe. Instead, scientific progression takes large periodic leaps. This fundamentally discredits positivism, as if there are large steps in human understanding there must be long periods during which false beliefs are held, based on previously existing sensory or experimental data.

The problems of positivism have not made the theory on which it is based less attractive. Indeed, it has been modified as these problems have arisen, and it is now supported as a verification principle; that is, only those thoughts and actions that can be verified against sensory data can be held to be true. As an extension of this principle, EBM looks at what could be termed the best verifiable clinical evidence available. Therefore, the beliefs of the past were the best evidence available, and are legitimate. This appears to be a somewhat circular argument.

In a recent review, Misak[1] indicated other important problems associated with the general adoption of the principle of the verification of facts against sensory data. She pointed to three major problems:

1. the restriction of language, in that it is only possible to ask questions about facts which can be verified
2. the assumption that verificationism makes about the ability of humans to practically demonstrate facts and perform tasks
3. problems associated with the sequential nature of human thought and action.

Each of these problems has a profound influence on the practice of evidence-based medicine and it is worthwhile considering each in greater detail.

The restriction of language

Under verificationist ideas questions can only be asked in such a manner that they can be verified. This demand explains why in the practice of EBM so much emphasis is placed on the way in which questions are asked. If questions are to be verifiable they must not have any metaphysical content; that is, they must not refer to abstract concepts such as pain – unless these ideas are related to a physical phenomenon, for example, the stimulation of C fibres. The difficulties positivism has with metaphysical ideas have a profound effect on EBM for they deny the existence of diseases of the mind. The inability to deal with the psychology of illness reverses a trend which has developed over the last few years for holistic medicine.

The use of verification questions based on sensory data brings with it other problems. If the development of medicine does not fit the incremental model of 'scientific' development then there is a mismatch between the questions asked and the facts available. Taking first, Kuhn's idea that the individual scientists and clinical perceptions play a major role in the shape of developments: where this is found to be true there may be a tendency for research to take place in the common condition where it is financially rewarding, or in the rare complex condition where it is professionally gratifying to conduct research. This theme has been explored in depth by Lyotard as the 'principle of performavity'.[5] This principle highlights the particular problems associated with the situation where information becomes allied to a commodity and when information becomes a utility in its own right. Lyotard's analysis suggests that if verification principles are applied there will be a tendency to produce answers to the common questions or the difficult questions only – regardless of patient suffering. This might lead to a utilitarian practice of medicine, in which the benefits of medical care are distributed in accordance with the greatest good for the greatest number.

The tendency towards utilitarianism under positivistic and empirical ideas is a common problem. John Stuart Mill, one of the founders of empiricist thought, used verification ideas to justify the use of utilitarianism.[6] Later still, the eugenists, such as Herbert Spencer, also used positivism and empirical arguments to justify the existence of racial supremacy.[7] It is not surprising that the suggestion that evidence-based medicine may lead to utilitarian-based decision-making leads to considerable concern in the medical and ethical research community.

Utilitarian ideas ignore all concept of relative human suffering and the 'right', as humans, to have that suffering relieved. In doing so, all concepts of equity are abandoned as it cuts across all of the moral boundaries in current society. The case of child B highlights the dilemma posed by utilitarian ideals. In this case the ruling of the judge permitted the health authority to withhold treatment of the child in view of the large number of potential benefactors that the money for the cancer treatment could assist. It is a paradox that although EBM starts with the benefit to the individual, the result – because of the nature of the evidence available – is the development of a utilitarian ideal.

Returning to our thread of the problems of verificational questions and the model of scientific progression; if we consider Popper's objection to the scientific model then another set of questions is raised. If we recall, Popper was concerned that once a verification question is formed, all occurrences of the phenomenon become linked to that question and act to confirm – without question – the original occurrence. This has the effect that the original question and resultant actions are always verified. As a result, scientific progression occurs only when there is sufficient deviation from the original thesis to cause its modification.

Popper's points are important in relation to the development of medical ideas. Medicine sits at the interface between social sciences and biological sciences. Many of the advances in medicine have social causes; the decline of tuberculosis for example has far more to do with the changes in living conditions than the treatments available. Scientific reports often ignore this and, as a result, place a strong attribution of the results of the interventions on the treatments used, often ignoring the social and political undertones. Under these conditions, future success also becomes attributed to the original treatment and a myth develops. This myth not only becomes the acceptable way to behave, but excludes all others. The result is that medical practice becomes 'cookbook', i.e. limited to the execution of recipes, and innovation is stifled.

The restriction of language creates a further problem. If language is restricted to the description and questions about the treatments of illness it becomes highly technical and beyond the comprehension of lay people. Information used to drive EBM is, by its nature, technical. It is written in the common language of medicine and involves statistical and technical procedures outside the grasp of 'lay' individuals. The interpretation of the evidence presented and the decisions made using it are also linked to the values of the professional involved. Therefore, unless carefully implemented, the practice of EBM leads to a re-enforcement of professional values and resource allocation; in short, a technocratic allocation system. This has the danger of reducing patient choice and removing the decision-making role of the patient. This effect is combined with the problems of a utilitarian bias, as discussed previously.

The combination of a technocratic-driven and utilitarian-biased resource allocation-making process results in the so-called 'rule utilitarianism' resource allocation system. This is the classical form of utilitarianism as proposed by Bentham.[8] Its roots lie in the application of jurisprudence to social ideas, and relies on the ideal of the benevolence of impartial spectators to distribute resources to maximize satisfaction, according to the rules of evidence. It has been argued that such impartial spectators do not exist in health care.

If verification questions are problematical, how can they be improved? First, we have argued that the current concept of asking verification questions is too restrictive. This infers that evidence-based questions are narrow and lead to self-verification. One way around this problem is to look at the reformulation of questions along the lines that Popper suggests. He advocated the development of questions that can be falsified – for only in falsification is there truth. Second, we have argued that a wider range of individuals needs to be involved in the EBM process if utilitarian ideals are not to emerge. These suggestions are going to be left here for a while, but returned to later in the book, once the other issues raised have been tackled.

The practical demonstration of facts and human performance

We have already commented on the problems that EBM pose for those of us who are not particularly computer-literate (see p. 28). However, as it relies, to one degree or another, on information systems, either in term of eliciting the information from the patient or from a computer, the human performance aspect of EBM is very important.

The formulation of the question to be answered is dependent upon the diagnostic ability of clinicians. We know this varies from day-to-day and between training periods. Therefore, EBM requires a level of competency that is uniform. This can only be brought about by accreditation. This is not an argument that we can enter into here, but it is a neglected element of the implementation of evidence-based medicine.

The subject of the human factor in EBM has two other dimensions that should be introduced here – namely, interpretation and belief. Evidence-based medicine – as we have already stated – has not focused on the implementation of its ideas; there is no link between verification and intention. The proponents of EBM often feel that the demonstration of facts is enough. However, it is intrinsic to humans that we know that facts can be distorted; for example, a straight stick appears bent if it is dipped into water.

Husserl[9] and other philosophers have interpreted the fact that humans have a tendency to believe sensory phenomena over all other information, as the belief in only those facts that are privately verified. This argument considerably weakens the strength of papers and articles. This thought system is known as phenomenology. Phenomenology provides an alternative to EBM in consensus decision-making, where by sharing our internal beliefs new systems can be generated. Consensus-based medicine is attaining some credibility in the United States where it is being presented as an alternative to the problems generated by EBM.

Returning to the problems faced by changing behaviour in relation to presented evidence, it is apparent that the causes of a change in behaviour are poorly understood. Degrees of what is known as cognitive dissonance are present among doctors and other health care professionals. Cognitive dissonance is the act of clinging to a belief when the evidence suggests that the belief is false. Medical training can result in a lot of the dissonance perceived. As health professionals, we are taught to believe our own interpretations, and that patients can be misleading. However, there is more to dissonance among doctors than this, as medical behaviour can be changed – the rising sales on new drugs are a testimony to this. Therefore, more work is needed on medical values in order to make change more likely.

The sequential nature of human action

As humans we act sequentially, taking an action then appraising the results. At each stage we apply values to the outcome, dependent on the previous action. Evidence-based medicine calls for us to set the values we apply before assessing the evidence. Such an approach is known as 'decisionism'. There are many problems associated with applying decisionism in clinical practice, but the greatest of these is the application of values before we see the patient. More of this problem will be covered in Part IV.

Summary

Evidence-based medicine is based on positivism; that is, the application of 'provable' facts to human behaviour. There is some doubt as to the applicability of this model to health care. In addition, the adoption of the principle of EBM leads medicine along the path of utilitarianism, or the greatest good for the greatest number. This leads to an ethical dilemma – what is more important – human suffering or the benefit society gains from health care?

In addition to the problems posed on an ethical front, there are also practical problems associated with the use of pre-assigned values in making decisions, and the ability to ask and verify the facts placed in front of us. These problems are reflected in the performance of EBM in relation to the allocation of resources and the management of health care.

References

1. Misak CJ (1995)*Verificationism*. Routledge, London.
2. Ayer AJ (1969) *Metaphysics and commonsense*. Macmillan, London.
3. Kuhn T (1970) *The structure of scientific revolutions*. University of Chicago Press, Chicago.

4. Popper K (1963) *Conjectures and refutations.* Routledge and Kegan Paul, London.
5. Lyotard JF (translated by G Bennington and B Massumi) (1979) *A post-modern condition.* Manchester University Press, Manchester.
6. Mill JS (1962) *Utilitarianism.* Fontana, London.
7. Spencer H (1843) *The proper sphere of government.* Pamphlet.
8. Bentham J (1962) In: JS Mill, *Utilitarianism.* Fontana, London.
9. Husserl E (1950) *Husserliania I.* The Hague.

7 Concerns about evidence-based medicine

> *Key points from the previous chapter*
>
> The development of evidence-based medicine from a positivistic creed suggests that in application it has positivistic tendencies. These, if followed, will lead to a practice of medicine that is utilitarian – a feature with strong ethical overtones. These overtones have a considerable impact on the management of health care and how resources are allocated within a limited health care budget.

This chapter reflects on the shortcomings in the philosophy of EBM; for while nobody would doubt the importance of giving the individual treatments that work, it should not overshadow the effects such a policy might have if the evidence is skewed. It features three areas: resource allocation, politics and management.

Background

The concerns about EBM are derived from the work of the Frankfurt school, who responded to the rise of rationalism in the mid-part of the twentieth century.[1] The Frankfurt school saw a rising trend in:

- the mathematical explanation of experience
- the extension of scientific practice into everyday life
- the application of ethical concepts to values which are determined before decisions are made – so-called fixed goal ethics.

They saw a danger, not in the application of these practices themselves, but in the resultant technocratic decision-making processes that developed from them. They characterized these processes as means-end rationality that resulted in:

- the reinforcement of professional values as to the distribution of welfare benefit
- the utilitarian processing of resource allocation
- rule-guided resource allocation without concern to suffering
- an alteration in the politics of welfare benefit.

In Chapter 6 we discussed the origins of these concerns; this chapter will discuss their impact.

Resource allocation

We have already discussed why EBM leads to utilitarianism, but why is the distribution of health care such that the 'greatest number' benefit such a bad thing?

In order to answer this question, first we must accept that it would be perfectly possible to conceive of a health care system based on utilitarian values. What would such a system look like? It would be selective in that not everybody would be treated. It would focus treatment on those with common diseases. This would have a paradoxical effect. While it implies there would be a focus on cardiovascular disease – which is a common illness – if the majority of a society were smokers then considerable effort would be applied to the treatment of smoking-related diseases – unless some countervailing force were to be applied.

In an attempt to solve these problems it has been suggested that doctors should put their individual response to the patient first and then use EBM to determine if the patient should access the care that is warranted by the disease.[2] This shifts the emphasis from evidence-based medicine on to evidence-based ethics. This change, which appears slight, has profound consequences on the future of EBM. First, the suggested change leads to an open admission of the ethical problems associated with

EBM. Second, the use of evidence to justify an ethical decision is dangerous as it could lead to the eugenic arguments as mentioned in Chapter 6. In short, it places a great deal of emphasis on the integrity of the doctor. In this situation, professional attitudes are key. If the professionals act as true advocates of the patient then they will impartially distribute benefits – as described in rule utilitarianism. However, as The Commission on Social Justice has demonstrated, this is not the case and patients are denied treatment on the professional's perception of the ability to benefit.[3] This 'ability' often includes social class, and in this manner EBM may increase the social disparities of medical care. A way out of this latter problem would be to involve the public in decision-making to a greater degree. However, this compromise runs against EBM as a technocratic process and has heavy political overtones.

Politics

The problems posed by resource allocation and EBM are in many ways exacerbated by the political problems faced by health care. Health has always been a political issue. This has been especially true in the twentieth century where a succession of changes has taken place regarding the political ideology of welfare in general. The early part still clung to the remnants of *laissez-faire*; that is, the role of the state was to control society in such a way that capital and industry were allowed to develop. In 1911 this was replaced by state-sponsored self-help, with the introduction of Lloyd George's insurance acts. The common thread across both of these ideologies is an emphasis on the role of the individual to secure their own welfare and the role of the state in being selective in the care it provides to those who need welfare support.

The selective elements of welfare were replaced during the Second World War by a universalist ideology as exemplified by the emergency medical service (EMS). Under this ideology, the state provided welfare for everybody, removing the need for the individual to secure a future if illness or unemployment struck. Since the mid 1960s this trend has reversed, in part due to the costs associated with a universal state, but also due to a change in ideology associated with the provision of welfare in these later years.

The change in political ideology can best be explained by a switch back to selective welfare services. Therefore welfare services are provided to 'those in need' rather than universally. It is tempting to associate this change with the latter Conservative governments, but the trend to selective services goes back much further to the 'civilized selectivity' of the Labour party in the 1960s. It is the trend for selectivity in health care that has added an acceptable element to evidence-based medicine.

Initial attempts at selectivity focused on selecting individuals. This policy – as we will see – has proved to be unpopular. In response to this, the selection by procedure – as proposed by EBM – appears to be a suitable alternative. In one sense, EBM is selective on the care it provides and therefore releases more resources to those in need. However, it calls into question the definition of those most in need.

The politics of need is a complex subject, and often ignored as a result. The discussions on human need are best covered in the work of Len Doyal.[4] He argues that need can be characterized as autonomy leading to social participation. Therefore on a personal level, need can be interpreted as desiring things and services to maximize the individual's role in society. It is argued by 'rights-based' sociologists that the relief of such needs is a basic right. However, as we have seen, the existence of EBM tends towards utilitarian-based ethics. Here it is not the degree of suffering but the number of individuals suffering which is a problem. Therefore the existence of EBM puts a different emphasis on the role of the selective political ideology; where selectivity of services drives the selectivity of those who benefit. This paradox is one of the biggest unsolved problems in evidence-based approaches.

The impact of the selectivity of services driving those who

will selectively benefit from health care has profound consequences for the interaction between society and the state. In many societies, health care is not a basic right to citizens – this includes the UK. It implies that despite making contributions to health care as part of the welfare scheme, patients will be denied benefit if no effective care can be found from which the patient will benefit. This change in the contract needs to be made explicit.

Whilst EBM provides a problem to the state/society definition, it does however solve a political problem. Politicians have sought to distance themselves from the political maelstrom associated with rationing, that is, in turn, associated with a selective health service based on individuals. Evidence-based medicine, with its emphasis on providing the greatest benefit for the greatest number, and while giving the power of rationing to the professionals, in effect, depoliticizes health care. The decisions that are made can be linked to professional values – it is only the total level of funds devoted to health care that is open for debate.

The combined impact of depoliticization and the change in the state/individual interaction influences what Habermas[5] has called the public sphere of health care; that is, it reduces the forum for rational debate about health care, both in terms of volume and in restricting those involved. While this restriction in the short term is advantageous to the political problems that surround health care, potentially it can do long-term damage, as it may serve to create powerful lobby groups and seek to increase the commodity value of information. This – as discussed later – will further distort the availability of health care away from those most in need.

Management

When the NHS was formed, the belief was that the provision of health care would reduce illness, therefore reducing demand. The belief had profound influence on the management of the service. The role of management was to ensure a smooth and steady supply of patients to the 'process' of medicine as practised by doctors, nurses and other professionals. In this way, the process of health care took place by managing surrogate markers of the process, such as waiting lists and finance. This belief was adhered to until the 1960s and early 1970s when the combination of demographic trends, technological expansion and the oil crisis, forced a rethink. These factors made it apparent that the demand for health care could well be infinite, whereas need for health care may not. This realization enforced a belief that medical care needed to be managed in such a way that needs were met, not demands.

With the advancement of medicine the proposition that needs are finite has also come under question. If needs are taken to mean acts that restore the individual back to a place in society, then the longer-living population will generate more needs. Therefore the totality of needs is also potentially infinite. For this reason, the emphasis of medical management in recent years has again shifted to the management of benefit. Initially it took the form of patient selection; the managerial idea behind the working of internal markets in health care. However, as we have discussed, the emphasis has recently shifted to management by procedure – the concept of evidence-based medicine.

The first endeavours at the management of health care services and process date back to the mid 1970s with the early attempts to produce programme budgets based on the demand for services. As we have seen, demand is potentially infinite and so these attempts failed. Is was not until the Thatcher government of the 1980s that the ideas of a truly selective health care service took shape. The Griffiths Report of 1983 was the first attempt to introduce a dedicated management structure, and 'need side' management of the process. However, the effectiveness of this approach could not be realized until the purchaser–provider split. The purchaser–provider split – also known as internal markets or quasi markets – provides a means to introduce choice and competition in health care. It enables the state-financed purchasers of health care to contract for a range of services from state and privately-owned providers of care; the tools of commercial management and economics are brought to bear on the health care process. In this system, financial levers and resource shifts become possible and the macro-management of the health care process achieves efficiencies at lower levels.

Health care process management has been bedevilled by claims that the transaction costs are too high and that it is ineffective. These claims are, in part, due to the politics that surround health, but there is also a truth to the accusations. The problem is caused by the lack of a core process to health care. In short, what is the purpose of health care? Is it to provide a health service or an illness service, for example. Evidence-based medicine goes a long way to providing that core as it firmly gives health care the purpose of restoring individuals to health, using evidence.

Taking these arguments, the role of health care management in the 1990s is to support the allocation of resources along evidence-based lines and in line with the political ideology of selectivity; that is, those who need the care should benefit most. Therefore the role of the manager in modern health care is that of a balancing act – balancing the restraints on care placed by evidence-based medicine against the pressure to help those most in need.

As if the role of tightrope walker is not enough, however, there are added complications. The measurement of how good a manager is at influencing selectivity is difficult and we have already commented on measuring how evidence-based is 'based on evidence' is impossible. In this situation, the counting of numbers treated is usually substituted. In the UK this is reflected in terms of the efficiency index – a calculation based on weighting activity. This favours hospital therapies over community care and has the effect of providing an incentive to treat patients in hospital, which in turn increases the amount of evidence-based care. Therefore, a self-feeding circle is established within which the quality of care is not measured.

The combination of the current performance indicators – as typified by the efficiency index – serves only to increase the technocratic allocation of resources, and reduce the flexibility and patient choice associated with the provision of a purchaser–provider split. It also decreases the power of the manager to intervene in the process of health care and ensure equity of resource distribution. In short, the process of EBM may be unmanageable in its current form.

In order to mitigate this effect, increasing interest is being shown in the micro-management of the health care process using initiatives such as managed care and disease management. These health care initiatives shift the emphasis away from the global management of health care into a series of tool-based assessments.

Disease management has been defined as a system of controls such that medical interventions focus on the provision of optimal health care to the patient. It uses:

- benefit restriction; in that only certain patients benefit from intervention based on need or severity of illness
- restrictions on physicians as to the services they can offer and the patients they can offer it to
- a system of variance reporting to control the flow of patients
- financial risk sharing to control the distribution of medical benefits.

It is a controversial subject and is gaining popularity in Europe in response to the failure of macro-management. However the use of evidence to underline its macro-tools has led some commentators to express concern over its effects on equity and justice – in a similar way to EBM, as explained above.

In response to the concerns about managed care, some effort is now being concentrated into involving the public in the management of medicine, particularly in the area of priority setting. However, these efforts are still under evaluation and we shall postpone discussing them until we have reviewed cost-effectiveness associated decision-making in medical practice.

Summary

Evidence-based medicine has consequences beyond the decisions about medical treatments. It has important political and managerial effects, which may make it untenable. However, it is important to stress that it is not EBM *per se* that is at fault, but its application in the current health system that provokes the issues.

This has led to increasing interest in managed care and disease management. However, these may only exacerbate the problems.

Part II summary

In Part II we have overviewed the history and development of evidence-based medicine and tried to relate it to the current medical and managerial environment.

Evidence-based medicine clearly has ramifications beyond that of medical management and an impact that spreads into politics, philosophy and ethics. Overall, nobody can deny that patients should receive effective and safe medicines; however, one of the difficulties that we have highlighted is the lack of definition as to what effective really means and whose effectiveness is to be considered. Ultimately, these problems cannot be solved easily without restructuring the way in which we look at medical practice. This will be dealt with in Part IV.

References

1. Held D (1980) *Introduction to critical theory*. Polity Press, Cambridge.
2. Sacklett D (1996) Evidence-based medicine, cost utility and the physician. Office of Health Economics talk, summarized in the *OHE News*.

3. The Commission on Social Justice (1994) *Strategies for national renewal.* Vintage, London.
4. Doyal L and Gough I (1991) *A theory of human need.* MacMillan, London.
5. Habermas J (1989) *The structural transformation of the public sphere.* Polity Press, Cambridge.

Part III Cost-effectiveness in Medicine

8 Cost-effectiveness in medical decision-making

Key points from previous chapters

The alternative model for medical decision-making is cost-effectiveness based decision-making, which is held to have a number of advantages over evidence-based medicine.

Cost is now an implicit part of every medical decision, and therefore cost-effectiveness based decision-making is part of the rationing debate. Cost-effectiveness based decision-making in medicine has different, but parallel aims to EBM, but also brings with it a new range of concerns and problems, all of which are discussed in this chapter.

An introduction to cost-effectiveness based medical decision-making (CEM)

What is cost-effectiveness?

'That's all well and good but is it cost-effective?' – a common enough question, but where does it come from and what does it mean? Simple statements often hide complex meanings – and so it is with CEM where 'lay' and professional vocabularies can often become confused and are then about as clear as a tax return.

Cost-effectiveness analysis is a branch of decision theory. Decision theory in its turn has been defined as 'the use of systematic methods for assessing the relative values of out-

51

comes'.[1] Within this definition a range of scenarios is possible. Value can be expressed in monetary or other terms, and outcomes likewise. Also, relative implies some ratio or chance of an event occurring.

The definition is so broad as to be useless. In usual practice it is applied to medicine as the aim of cost-effectiveness associated medical decision-making is to 'maximize the benefit to patients, given the constraints of scarce resources'.[1]

This aim brings CEM into contrast with EBM-based decisions. CEM concerns itself with relative values for populations of patients, while EBM is concerned with absolute benefit to the individual. From the outset CEM is, by nature, concerned with utilitarian values in seeking maximal benefit for a group of individuals. Therefore it is immediately subject to the ethical concerns about utilitarianism discussed in the previous chapter. However, the hope is that in this explicitness the distortion can be accounted for.

As was mentioned above, the foundation of CEM lies in decision theory, a technique first developed in relation to the oil industry in the 1950s. Decision analysis is a group of associated techniques that tries to express the relative value of an outcome or event in terms of the magnitude achieved and the probability of that maximum actually occurring. One of these tools is cost-effectiveness analysis where the relative values are expressed in monetary terms. CEM is a direct development of cost-effectiveness analysis. In CEM therefore the important values considered are the costs of the intervention, the magnitude of the treatment effects and the probabilities that the desired effects will be achieved.

Decision analysis has a long history in medicine. Early efforts focused on the development of diagnostic and treatment pathways, but in recent years there has been a renewed interest in using costs to determine the relative value of outcomes. This in turn has spawned the interest in cost-effectiveness analysis in medical decision-making. In this situation, cost-effectiveness analysis is of most value in policy-making in complex situations involving decisions across time and where information is uncertain.

Although the focus on relative value makes the process of analysis somewhat different, CEM has a great many similarities to EBM. First, they are empiricist in that both EBM and CEM have a foundation in the demonstration of benefit to patients. Second, they are decisionist in that they rely on the predetermination of the values that are applied to the decision being determined, before the decision is taken. Therefore in some ways CEM suffers from the same problems and concerns as those seen in EBM – a point we will return to. However, CEM does have the advantage that a wider range of values can be inserted into decisions, as we will explore later.

Cost-effectiveness based medical decision-making is a development of industrial decision theory in which the costs and relative outcomes of an intervention are considered. The application of CEM immediately implies an ethical dilemma as the benefits for populations are being examined.

Reference

1. Pettiti DB (1994) *Meta-analysis, decision analysis and cost-effectiveness analysis.* Oxford University Press, Oxford.

9 The process of cost-effectiveness analysis in medical decision-making

> **Key points from the previous chapter**
>
> *The process of CEM involves the demonstration of the relative value of decision options using cost-effectiveness analysis as a basis. It does this by means of a standardized process which looks at maximizing benefits to populations, however these benefits may be demonstrated.*

Cost-effectiveness analysis follows a process similar to EBM. This chapter overviews these major points and introduces some crucial issues.

In order to explain the principles let us consider the example of the eradication of *Helicobacter pylori* – the accepted cause of gastric ulcer disease.[1]

Background

Helicobacter pylori is a recently-identified cause of gastric ulceration. Almost all patients who have gastric ulcers not associated with drugs such as aspirin are positive for the organism. A course of therapy designed to eradicate the organism is successful in curing the ulcer. However, a significant number of individuals are also positive for the organisms but negative for ulcers.

Identification and bounding of the problem

The first part of a cost-effectiveness analysis is to identify and bound the problem. The objective of this stage is to develop a concise statement that identifies all the relevant issues in the question. This step has parallels to asking questions in EBM. A suitable question might be: 'Is the screening for, and eradication of, *Helicobacter pylori* cost-effective in men under 45 years of age?'.

As part of the identification of the question, the recognition of alternatives is important. In our example it is easy − to screen or not to screen. It is not always that simple. In general the selection of alternatives must:

- be ethical
- be representative of current practice
- represent complete episodes of treatment.

All too often, the selection of alternatives is poorly performed and inappropriate. This not only weakens the result but discredits it with the readers of such papers.

Once the question and the alternatives are established, the boundaries are located. This involves the setting of the inputs and outcomes. In our example, the input is the cost of screening and the outcome the eradication of the causative organism. The boundaries of these inputs and outcomes are expressed in financial terms in the cost of screening and eradication therapy. However, it should be borne in mind that other expressions are possible.

The outcome of cost-effectiveness analysis in health care can be expressed in a variety of ways. The nature of the outcome selected on the whole sets the terms of the analysis. If outcomes are expressed in terms of monetary value then it is a form of cost−benefit analysis. This is not the usual type featured. Instead, others are favoured. The advantage of cost−benefit analysis is that seemingly unconnected options can be compared; for example, a comparison of the benefits of hospital versus road building. Perhaps it is this diversity that makes cost–benefit analysis so distasteful.

Cost–benefit analysis has been criticized as it places a value on human life and the financial consequences of health care may be hard to identify. In its place other types of analysis have been suggested. These include:

- measuring the outcome of treatment in terms of natural units, e.g. years of life saved or decline in blood pressure. This approach has been criticized as it is difficult to tell if a meaningful result has been achieved. Do patients want more life? This approach has been termed – confusingly – cost-effectiveness analysis

- a measure of satisfaction with the treatment given – often termed utility measures. Utility measures include some aspects of quality of life measurement and synthetic measures such as quality adjusted life years (QALYs). More will be said of these measures later.

- patient-based values. One of the major attractions of the use of CEM is to incorporate patient values outside the satisfaction with treatment; for example, a population preference for the distribution of resources. It is increasingly apparent that patient choice is becoming a major factor as choice increases. Patient values can be included in one of two ways. First, patient values can be used to adjust the probabilities of outcomes being achieved. This is usually done by the formation of consensus groups. The second approach is to use patient-defined outcomes. An example of this approach is the use of lifetime goals in asthma. A great deal of interest is being shown in these methods; however their diversity appears to rule out a role in medical decision-making.

The incorporation of patient values raises a number of practical issues. First, patient preferences must be elicited in a semi-independent manner: too much structure and a subgroup will dominate, too little and there will be as many opinions as participants plus one. The second problem concerns how to express the results. This is part of a much wider issue that incorporates the problems of utility measures that were alluded to above.

A utility measure is an outcome that encompasses the satisfaction with or preference for a medical state after treatment. There are a variety of ways in which these preferences can be expressed. They can be determined by the use of direct measurement scales; for example, questionnaires or visual analogue scales. Alternatively they can be measured by looking at the value of time spent in a state as opposed to full health – the so-called time trade-off methods. However the preferences are measured it should be realized that these methods are very sensitive to the perception of the person who is being scored and the way in which the questions are asked. For example, consider two groups of students who are faced with two choices for the management of a hypothetical disease that attacks 600 patients each year.

Group A
Choice 1 – 200 lives will be saved
Choice 2 – 0.33 chance that 600 lives will be saved
Group B
Choice 1 – 400 lives will be lost
Choice 2 – 0.33 chance of no fatalities

Experimentally, Group A chose 1 and Group B chose 2. However, in reality there is no difference between any of the options presented. Therefore language and presentation play a major role in determining the utility of health care.

Another aspect of the bounding of the analysis is setting the perspective. The costs of procedures vary greatly, depending on how they are viewed; e.g. the cost of a hospital stay to a provider is reflected in the charges for the bed (but is not identical to the charges as these include, for example, profit margins). However, for a patient it may be reflected in the time they spend off work. It is important, therefore, to state explicitly how the analysis is being viewed. In the case of the *H. pylori* problem we are using the purchaser perspective so that the cost is all that matters. Increasingly, the perspective is being viewed as society's, so that all costs and benefits are included.

Structuring the problem

The bounded problem is expressed symbolically as a decision tree. A decision tree is a right to left assemblage of nodes representing the decisions and outcomes. The example of our problem is shown in Figure 9.1. A decision node is a point where a decision is made between competing alternatives, e.g. where a choice is made to screen or not. A chance node represents where an outcome that can occur is probability-dependent, e.g. the chances of screening being positive. An outcome node represents the result of the final outcome of the decision and the chance.

The structuring of the problem is key to the solution. However, it is possible to see that with more than one outcome and several treatments the problem structures can become very complex. An alternative way to look at the problem is to use techniques such as Markov models, where the outcomes are expressed as a series of disease states, such as well, mobile, dead, etc. The patient then transits between these states in a time- and probability-dependent manner. The use of Markov models requires specialized mathematical knowledge, beyond the scope of this text. The interested reader is referred to the Further reading list at the end of the chapter.

Gathering information

Once the tree, or Markov model, is constructed then information is gathered to populate it. Information can be obtained from a variety of sources, for example:

- the meta-analysis of studies
- clinical trials
- expert or consensus information
- hospital cost records.

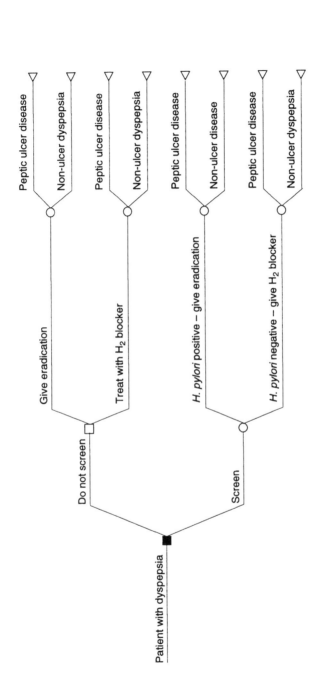

Figure 9.1 Basic decision tree based on the clinical problem.

The collection of cost data is often the most difficult part. It is important to differentiate costs from charges and to understand that it is economic cost that interests the analysis. Strictly speaking, it is economic cost that is relevant to the analysis, i.e. the value of the benefit forgone, but this is not possible in medical practice. Instead three cost categories are substituted. These are:

1. direct costs – i.e. the costs associated directly with the treatment of disease
2. indirect costs – i.e. the costs associated with the lost production to society
3. intangible costs – i.e. the costs of suffering to the patients and their carers.

The costs involved in an analysis depend very much on the perspective of the analysis. For example, indirect costs do not matter if the analysis is purely from the hospital viewpoint. However, indirect costs may dwarf direct costs – especially where domiciliary care for chronic diseases is concerned. It is vital in any analysis that all costs are considered appropriately.

The collection of cost data is also a problem. In countries with a private health service cost data may be obtainable from the insurers – but largely for direct costs only. In many cases we are left substituting an imputed market value for the costs of nursing time and care-giver time. Intangible costs are, at present, almost impossible to calculate accurately.

The incorporation of information into the decision tree is often the most difficult part. The data we have included in our tree has to be extracted from the information given in the article. Hence: the estimate of the number of dyspeptic patients with *H. pylori* infection is said to be 40%. Therefore a patient with dyspepsia has a 0.4 probability that they are infected with the organism. However, the probability of success must be calculated by multiplying the overall success rate by the probability that the dyspeptic patient is positive for the causal organism. Here we reach a critical point, for in this analysis we have chosen to ignore any non-specific tests.

Like the outcome results, the costs are also estimated from the paper. We therefore assume that the costs of eradication is £40; testing, £50: H_2 blocker (the alternative medication) is £50 per year. All of these figures are incorporated into the tree with the financial details being displayed on the right-hand side. The completed tree is shown in Figure 9.2.

Analysing the tree

As we stated above the tree is analysed – or rolled back in tree parlance – by multiplying the probability by the financial outcomes. This is shown in Figure 9.3. In this case, the computer program used has identified the best pathway based on the lowest cost: not to screen and to treat with H_2 blockers will result in the lowest cost.

Sensitivity analysis

The power of decision analysis lies in its capacity to handle uncertain information. This is accomplished in part by using the estimates of probabilities, but also by the use of sensitivity analysis. The development of the model structure involves making assumptions about key variables. During the sensitivity analysis these assumptions are tested by varying them and looking at the overall effect on the tree that has been built. For example, we could vary the costs by 10% or change the probabilities of success by a similar amount and re-run the table. In our example, no changes tried within these ranges affected the final result – therefore the tree is insensitive to change. If changes to the final pathway chosen did occur then it would be important to quantify the changes and to look at how real the assumptions were. An explicate sensitivity analysis is an important part of an analysis.

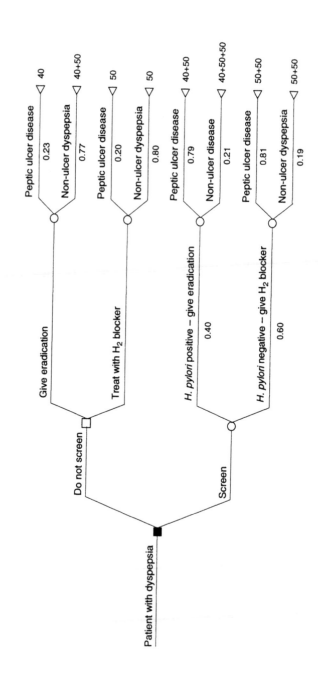

Figure 9.2 Decision tree after addition of probabilities and costs.

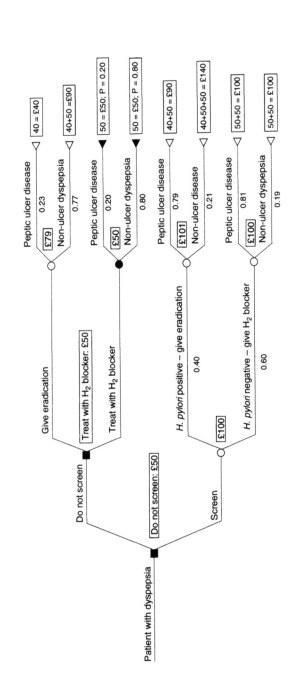

Figure 9.3 The rolled back decision tree for *H. pylori* problem.

Discounting

The construction and analysis of a decision tree often involves the comparison of costs and benefits that occur in different time periods. If this is so then these different periods must be accounted for by discounting.

Discounting is a factor of human nature, not economics. It is not related directly to inflation, although the level of inflation does impact the interest rate, which is discounting in reverse. Discounting takes into account the time value of money; that is, money now is perceived to be worth more than the same money in the future. Discounting can also be applied to benefits in a similar manner. Discounting is one of the most complex issues raised in decision analysis and there is little agreement on how it should be applied.

In setting the discount rate it is customary to set a rate close to the prevailing interest rate, but then to perform a sensitivity analysis around it. The currently accepted rate is about 6%. All costs and benefits occurring outside the base year are then reduced by a factor proportional to the rate. For example, if the treatment with H_2 blocker therapy in our *H. pylori* example was for more than a year, the first year would cost £50, but the second would be valued at £50 minus 6%, or £47. The discount effect is quite important, therefore, in time-dependent events.

Reporting the results

In reporting the results, the graphical representation – in the form of the tree – and the results are required. In presenting the results of the analysis, consideration needs to be given to whether the results are to be presented incrementally or in totality. Incremental analysis expresses the cost-effectiveness of the alternatives as a ratio. It is defined as the cost-per-unit effectiveness as a result of switching from one treatment to another, or preferring one treatment over another. Therefore:

$$\text{incremental cost-effectiveness} = \frac{\text{difference in cost}}{\text{difference in effectiveness}}$$

where

difference in cost = cost of intervention – cost of alternative

and

$$\text{difference in effectiveness} =$$
effectiveness of intervention – effectiveness of alternative.

The incremental cost-effectiveness is often confused with the average cost-effectiveness which is:

$$\text{average cost-effectiveness} = \frac{\text{total cost}}{\text{total effect}}$$

The average cost-effectiveness is misleading as it is non-comparative and therefore useless in making a medical decision. Whenever possible, results should be presented as an incremental cost-effectiveness ratio. In addition to the incremental report, a review of the assumptions made, sensitivity analysis and perspectives used are also mandatory. Finally, it should be remembered that the aim of the report is to be useful, not to blind people completely!

Summary

Cost-effectiveness analysis is a process for demonstrating the potential relative value of alternative medical interventions. This process includes:

- identification and bounding of the problem
- constructing a decision tree or other model
- gathering the data to fill the model
- analysis
- sensitivity analysis
- discounting
- reporting.

The aim of the analysis is to produce a measure of the programme's cost-effectiveness – usually presented as an incremental cost-effectiveness ratio.

Reference

1. Briggs AH, Sculpher MJ, Logan RP *et al.* (1996) Cost effectiveness of screening for and eradication of *Helicobacter pylori* in management of dyspeptic patients under 45 years of age. *BMJ*. **312**: 1321–5.

Further reading

Petitti DB (1994) *Meta-analysis, decision analysis and cost-effectiveness analysis.* Oxford University Press, Oxford.

10 The effects of cost-effectiveness based medical decision-making

> *Key points from the previous chapter*
>
> *Cost-effectiveness based medical decision-making (CEM) is a process for comparing the relative value of health care interventions. It relies on a set process for developing the result – usually expressed as an incremental cost ratio – which is derived from the performance of a decision analysis.*

Like evidence-based medicine, CEM has evolved into an industry – but what has it done for the practitioners and recipients of medical care? This chapter reviews its effects.

How important is CEM?

It would not be an over-exaggeration to say that at least once a month every journal has an article on CEM. This implies very clearly that there is a belief that the information provided is important to somebody – the question is, who? When the phenomenon of the publication explosion is looked at, however, a different picture emerges. First, there is confusion about what CEM is, and then there is a wide interpretation of the process. In some articles consideration is given to direct cost alone without discussion of outcomes. These analyses – so common that the term *cost minimization* has been invented to cover them – often give little or no justification for the assumption that underlies these techniques, namely that the alternatives compared are equally effective. While these analyses may be valid they instil a sense of distrust.

Yet there is a demand for genuine information. Many surveys of hospital staff and general practitioners place the inclusion of information on cost-effectiveness very high on their wish list. On the down side of these surveys, however, is the apparent distrust of information generated by the pharmaceutical companies and reports that the information provided is quite often difficult to understand.

The problems with the credibility and understanding of CEM information have direct parallels to the situation discussed in evidence-based medicine. Therefore, for CEM to have an impact, considerable thought must be given to reviewing how we ask questions, and how we identify and bound problems. Reviews of the effects of CEM have also – like in EBM – pointed to the time constraints imposed by it on retrieving information. In addition, these reviews also point to other problems in the use of cost-effectiveness information in medical care.

Medical care is now very diverse, in terms of its remit, technology, and its purpose and control. Each of these diversities causes a difficulty in the application of CEM. Underlying these difficulties – and in many ways magnifying them – are the dilemmas facing health care workers as a result of the purchaser–provider relationships seen across Europe. In many ways the development of purchaser–provider relationships is the reason why there is such a demand for CEM. Purchaser–provider splits – also called internal or quasi-markets – are an attempt to harness the power of economics into medical decision-making. Cost-effectiveness analysis relies on the assumptions underlining economics in order to produce valid conclusions. Two of these assumptions are of particular interest to us here. First, consumers have complete information about the things they are buying. Second, consumers are able to make choices based on both the information and their preference. These two assumptions underlying market mechanisms are very difficult to sustain in health care and lead to difficulty in applying CEM. The interaction occurs at the levels of the following.

Diversity of remit

Health care is expanding, not just in the technological sense but also in the range of services it encompasses. In many instances aspects of social and holistic care are now coming into medical and clinical practice. This leaves holes in the information available which reduce the ability of health care staff to make choices.

Diversity of technology

Technology is increasing at a rapid pace, and it is estimated that the body of knowledge is doubled every five years. Given this situation it is unlikely that information can ever be complete.

Diversity of purpose and control

Cost-effectiveness based medical decision-making makes an assumption that the purpose of health care structures is to provide efficient health care. However – again drawing parallels with EBM – this assumption is not altogether clear. Health care purchasers have other pressures to contend with and the purpose of providing efficient health care often becomes lost in a morass of performance management, public and media pressures. It is difficult to incorporate these values into CEM techniques as they are not outcomes in the usual sense. It is difficult to evaluate, for example, the effects of a performance measure on public perception. In this situation the information provided can only be an aid to decision-making.

Given these problems it is perhaps not surprising that in reviews of the impact of CEM it is suggested that CEM is of little value in deciding how resources should be spread across disease areas; for example, how much money should be spent on heart disease versus mental health. However, CEM is of much greater value in deciding how heart disease should be managed – but it is not the overriding factor.

Summary

CEM has not had the impact the pundits predicted, due for the most part to the complexity of health care in the modern world. What studies have been performed suggest that the information generated is of use in deciding priorities within disease groups not across them. However, as with EBM, there are problems in obtaining the information, and with its credibility.

Further reading

Honigsbaum F, Richards J and Lockett T (1995) *Priority setting in action: purchasing dilemmas.* Radcliffe Medical Press, Oxford.

11 Concerns about CEM and its future development

> *Key points from the previous chapter*
>
> *Cost-effectiveness based medical decision-making has not been associated with changing practice due to the complexity of medical decisions. Particular complicating factors include the role of performance management and the increasing diversity of medical practice.*

Faced with the continuing pressure on health care expenditure, CEM is here to stay. However, it clearly needs some modification in view of the difficulties in adoption of the methods. This need for change is coupled with the need to link CEM to EBM, as EBM is now a significant – if changing movement. In addition, several concerns have been raised about the effects that CEM might have on resource allocation. This chapter reviews these concerns and looks at how CEM is developing.

Concerns about CEM

Concerns about CEM arise on two levels. First there are a range of concerns associated with the positivistic and decisionistic methods such as EBM and CEM. These were covered in the last section but to recap; the application of positivistic methods to health care gives rise to concern due to the impact these methods have on the justice of health care. They tend towards a utilitarian resource allocation with technocratic overtones. This leads to an enforcement of professional values and unless these are tempered by neutral advocates, human suffering may be ignored. The use of systems such as CEM and EBM also leads to situations where the values applied to a decision are decided upon before the patient is seen. This may not be compatible with the gatekeeper model of medical practice as is currently being developed. Finally, EBM and CEM may rely on a hypothesis about the generation of medical knowledge that is false, in that it assumes a smooth progression. This may not be the case and a stepwise or falsificationist progression is more likely. The effect of this misconception may be that innovation is stifled. From these postulates it is apparent that CEM, like EBM, is also linked to the managerialism and depoliticization of health care, with its inherent dangers.

The second concern about the use of CEM arises as a result of the incomplete nature of the internal market which the information is used to drive. As explained above, CEM is used in the context of the purchaser–provider split. For this to work well, complete information and preference determination is required. Where this situation does not prevail three results are possible:

1. *Market failure.* It is possible that markets could overheat as a result of misconceptions of value or the accuracy of information. If, for example, the cost-effectiveness of a procedure is overestimated, then investment will be lost and deficits accrue. Some evidence for this has already been seen in situations where the prices of services were accepted to be completely accurate.
2. *Moral hazard.* Where the distribution of information is unbalanced, for example, where a provider knows their specific costs to be higher than those included in the cost-effectiveness analysis, then there is the potential for exploitation of the imbalance – so-called moral hazard. If acute, this will lead to forms of market failure.

The above two concerns will lead to the total collapse of the health care system – affecting all individuals equally. However, there is a third concern which is more subtle and leads to injustice.

3. If CEM information is not uniformly developed then there is the risk that a focus on a population may develop such that funds are diverted away from the most needy. For example, it is known that grommets are not effective in the majority of children with glue ear, but the population with glue ear tends to be from lower social classes. If funds are withdrawn on the basis of CEM then they may be used to purchase other health care and spread over all social-class groups. The net result is a lowering of expenditure on the group that needs it most. CEM therefore argues for the creation of ring-fencing within the internal market to maintain justice in health care expenditure.

The development of CEM

The existence of the problems associated with both EBM and CEM argues for a review of the effects and attempts to mitigate the problems. The problems of utilitarian decision-making have now come to the notice of the medical profession and ways are being sought to moderate them. Accordingly, we are witnessing the bringing together of EBM and CEM in an attempt to unify question-making and identification. We also see uncertainty being introduced into EBM. However, these moves still keep benefit and cost as separate entities. Thought must be given to how best to consider these together with the justice of health care. This will be covered in the next chapter.

In an attempt to develop CEM further, another suggestion has been to develop to a greater extent the outcomes incorporated into the structure of the cost-effectiveness analysis. There have been suggestions that political outcomes should be included, but this approach has not received much support as they are often related to the party in question and are probably not acceptable to most clinicians. At present, outcomes tend to be unidimensional, for example, death or cure. Another approach, of increasing interest, is to incorporate the use of multidimensional (reflecting both clinical and process) outcomes; for example, the development of the so-called health compass (Figure 11.1). On the health compass four dimensions of outcome are recognized: cost, function, satisfaction and clinical.

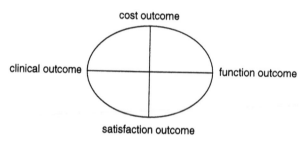

Figure 11.1 The health compass.

The compass approach defines the outcomes of CEM in disease states and looks to shift the emphasis towards the most important outcome in each disease. It also helps to decide if the outcomes to be measured are process-orientated, for example, cost or clinical, or focused (e.g. clinical outcome), or person orientated (e.g. functional outcomes). The decision about the major outcome enables the direction of the CEM to be determined.

Another way of defining multidimensional outcomes is the use of willingness-to-pay analysis. In this form of analysis, recipients of treatments are asked to value the care they have received in monetary terms. It is gaining in popularity but is still faced with considerable methodological problems.

As an alternative to using multidimensional outcomes, there is a move to develop representation of multiple outcomes on the same structure. An example of this is the more extensive use of models – such as Markov modelling and Monte Carlo simulations of processes.[1] These models are very complex and difficult to understand and use. It is the complexity that is their major disadvantage to acceptance and credibility.

Summary

CEM is associated with concerns about utilitarianism and market failure. These concerns are, on the whole, parallel to those seen in EBM. In response to these problems, amendments to the process of CEM are proposed. These amendments include:

- the unification of CEM and EBM
- the development of multidimensional outcomes
- the development of more complex models.

However, there is a considerable number of barriers to increasing the complexity of the analysis. Instead, effort is being focused on the development of different techniques – covered in Part IV.

Reference

1. Petitti DB (1994) *Meta-analysis, decision analysis and cost-effectiveness analysis.* Oxford University Press, Oxford.

Part IV Conclusion

12 So what matters, cost or benefit?

Key points from Parts I to III

There are two predominant forms of decision-making frameworks currently being applied in the present health care environment. These are evidence-based medicine and cost-effectiveness based medical decision-making. Both of these techniques have been borrowed from other disciplines and adapted to medical practice.

Evidence-based medicine seeks to maximize benefit to an individual patient, or at least minimize the harm caused by medical treatment. In contrast, cost-effectiveness based medical decision-making seeks to examine the relative values in monetary terms, of interventions and to use this information to provide maximum benefit to a population under conditions where resources are scarce.

As discussed in Parts I to III, both of these techniques have tendencies to produce positivism-based decision-making, which has a technocratic bias. This effect is mainly due to the nature of the information available and its impact leads to a utilitarian bias which may, in turn, lead to a shift of resources away from those most in need.

EBM and CEM are also in conflict. The application of EBM may increase the costs of medical practice. Therefore, a choice has to be made about which system of decision-making to apply.

This chapter explores the issues that surround the choices that must be made between EBM and CEM. In addition it provides alternative choices for consideration.

Cost or benefit?

The obvious answer is it depends – but depends on what? One of the catchphrases of modern health care is 'making the most of scarce resources'. In a sense, choosing the decision-making process depends on just this principle and both CEM and EBM will certainly fulfil the aim of making the best of available resources. They will act to increase the efficiency with which resources are consumed, by eliminating the use of ineffective treatments. However, as we have discussed, EBM may also demand new resources, by demonstrating a wider range of patient benefits. Therefore, in making a choice between CEM and EBM the perspective of the decision-maker becomes important. It is likely that those individuals concerned with the financing of health care will be attracted to cost–benefit arguments while the medical profession will be attracted to EBM. However, the question on perspective brings into view the potential for benefit for both the decision-making and the patients who are receiving treatment. In particular, it begs the question what are we trying to achieve with health care?

There are several views on the role of health care. Most societies agree to the need to provide some form of health care, although the way in which that care is provided varies from private finance to state taxation. Reasons why a society organizes health care include:

- maximization of productivity
- prevention of social unrest
- prevention of illness and suffering
- enabling those who are ill to return to normal health.

They key feature of all the reasons behind establishing health care organizations is the concept of selectivity. Health services are selective: they select individuals who have paid contributions to care, who need care or who demand care. But is this selectivity fair? This is embodied in the concept of equity.

Equity is a term that is hard to define, but it can be likened to the fairness of distribution of health care benefits. It is possible to consider this fairness in a number of dimensions, for example:

- fairness in access to health care
- fairness of opportunity to receive health care
- fairness of health status
- fairness of treatment.

The question, then, is not what matters – cost or benefit – but when do they matter, under the condition of who benefits. As an example, if the health care system is directed towards productivity, then the treatment of minor, non-productivity threatening illnesses can be considered on a cost basis alone. This approach is not a sterile one. In the case of a child with relapsing leukaemia, the life of that child can be valued above other interventions – so decisions about resource allocation in relation to who benefits are already being taken.

Decision-making by consideration of whom will benefit clearly has some problems. First, it immediately brings to mind the problem of deciding what a health service is for. Politicians, clinicians and the public will all have different ideas as to what the health care services should be achieving. The answer to this problem is not one-sided health care reforms – there is a need for an informed debate about health care itself. Second, the consideration of equity forces a more fundamental rethink about the types of information needed to decide health care resource allocation. In particular:

The widening of the concept of benefit

The current concept of benefit is often limited to the clinical benefit; for example, absolute blood pressure drops as a result of antihypertensive therapy. If evidence is to have a role in determining resource allocation then the concept needs to be widened considerably, and in two directions.

First, a consideration outside of clinical benefit into social and lifestyle benefits needs to occur. The improvement of a peak flow means little in the context of an asthmatic bed-bound by multiple sclerosis – an extreme example, but a rational one. The problem with widening the concept of evidence in this manner is that it weakens the power of the outcome measured in decision-making. A personal goal as an outcome, for example, is very little use in deciding if more resources are to be spent, unless it is united with some measure of the value of the benefit by looking at who benefits. The value of benefits to an individual in the context of a society is a controversial subject and underlines the need for bilateral health reforms, i.e. reforms not just of delivery systems but of the expectations of those who receive care. An example of this type of approach is the *Contract with America* proposed by Newt Gingrich, Speaker of the House of Representatives.

The widening of the concept of cost

Currently, too many approaches look at simple costs. PACT (a database held by the Department of Health on prescribing) and PRODIGY (decision-support software) in the UK are prime examples. All too often, the simple costs used are limited to mostly the acquisition costs. If the benefits of outcomes need redefinition to be of value in a who-benefits resource allocation system then so do the costs. The major advancement required in the use of costs in decision-making is an understanding of opportunity costs in health care. What is good value in health care compared to all of the complexities of modern living?

The proposals to adopt health funds are an example of attempts to harness the power of consumers' opportunity costs. Health funds, i.e. personally allocated sums of money to an individual with which they may choose to buy health care allows consumers to weigh-up individual costs and benefits so that the opportunity cost of one treatment can be compared with another. The use of health funds, however, is made complex by the calculations required to develop the fund sizes. An alternative is the voucher system of health care.

Neither of these two proposals addresses the issues of social costs. The assessment of costs to society requires an understanding of how society values the effect of health care to an individual, depending on the position of the individual within the society. This is clearly a difficult – but not impossible – task. Indeed, in the area of environmental economics it is common to carry out such appraisals using willingness-to-pay and other methods.

Internal markets

Spilling over from the concepts of costs and benefits is the use of competitive solutions to health care problems. It should be remembered that 'there are no normative solutions to health care markets' (Ali McQuire, 1995. Personal communication).

Traditional concepts of market efficiency and the evidence to drive it rely on the existence of equilibrium and other stable points in the market to determine good versus bad decisions. However, in internal markets there is no such equilibrium and good and bad must be viewed as personal value-based decisions. For this reason, health economics can only be a tool to aid decision-making. Therefore the value of cost-effectiveness information is always limited. However, the situation can be improved by the use of cost–benefit analyses. These analyses, which value both costs and benefits in monetary terms, permit the easier comparison of options across groups of individuals, and by the use of willingness-to-pay, can incorporate the individual values of patients. However, as mentioned previously, they are distasteful to some individuals because of the value they place on human life.

Ultimately, the use of competitive methods such as internal markets in allocating health care resources may lead to the adoption of utilitarian resource allocation if it remains unfettered. The easiest way in which the problems associated with markets may be solved is by the involvement of the public in decision-making.

Involving the public

The only decision-makers able to decide what is good for them are the public. In the final analysis, only the owners of the system can make the decisions about when benefit and cost matter. However, how to involve them is a difficult question. The public represents a kedgeree of different opinions, intellects and pressure groups. Many professionals doubt the ability of the public to make decisions; but ways are being found. The use of citizens' juries in the UK and other parts of Europe may provide a way forward, as may the spread of information technology, such as the Internet.

The involvement of the public provides the only counterbalance to the tendency to politicize health in an unhelpful way. However, involvement of the public will place an increased emphasis on expanding the concepts of benefit and cost, as the public view these ideas in a different way to the professional staff.

Expanding the evidence

Medical knowledge provides only a small part of the health care of a patient. Many inputs relating to health care come from nursing, social services, public health and environmental services, and education – to name but a few. Therefore, the concept of evidence-based medicine is in need of expansion to cover these areas.

Improving the presentation of, and access to, information

One of the keys to making the choice between cost and benefit is the availability of information and the way in which it is presented. We have already emphasized how positivistic methods reduce the linguistic content of questions – and how this is not always a good thing.

The language of medicine is a neglected subject, yet if decisions between cost and benefit are to be made then it is a subject worthy of further consideration. Coupled with this is access to the required information via more user friendly systems.

Pulling it all together

The choice between when to apply cost criteria and when to apply benefit involves the description of a purposeful system. This is an attempt to harness the underlying values of a system without always articulating them. The system therefore draws on both linguistic and social theories to disentangle norms from facts. It relies on a clear sense of purpose of the health care system – something not always present.

Conclusion

Both cost-effectiveness analysis and evidence-based medicine will not solve the problems of rationing and resource allocation, as in themselves they may exacerbate the problems. Instead it is requisite that rationing is determined by knowing when to apply evidence-based rules and when to apply cost-based rules. The decision to prioritize health care resources in this manner implies that a consideration of whom benefits are for, is needed.

If the allocation of resources is to consider individuals' benefit in health care, then some expansion of the concepts of both cost and benefit is required. However, the largest task is to establish the purpose of health care systems.

Index